Management in the acute ward

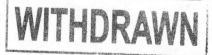

Key Management Skills in Nursing

Series editors Roswyn A Brown and George Castledine

Other titles in this series:

Dementia: management for nurses and community care workers *by Dr I B McIntosh and K Woodall*

Managing Continuing Education: A consumer's and provider's point of view *by Marilyn Williams*

Managing the Ethical Process in Research *by Marilyn Hammick*

Key Management Skills in Nursing

edited by
Roswyn A Brown and George Castledine

Management in the acute ward

by Jane Walton and Maggie Reeves

Quay
Books

Quay Books, Division of Mark Allen Publishing Limited
Jesses Farm, Snow Hill
Dinton, Nr Salisbury, Wilts, SP3 5HN, United Kingdom

©Mark Allen Publishing Limited, 1996
British Library Cataloguing-in-Publication Data
A catalogue record for this book is available from the British Library

ISBN 1-85642-041-8

Printed in the UK by Biddles Ltd, Guildford and King's Lynn

Contents

Chapter		Page.
Foreword		vii
Acknowledgements		viii
Introduction		ix
1.	Management of self and implications for the acute ward, including:-	1
	time management	5
	values	7
	leadership style	12
2.	Management of others which includes looking at aspects of:-	19
	being competent with management responsibilities concerning:-	21
	rules and regulations	25
	ward philosophy	26
	being a controller	27
	being an able communicator	28
	a negotiator with responsibility	33
	being a planner	35
	aware of the ward strategy	40
	being a decision maker	44
	a delegator	45
	being an implementor	45
	a motivator and organisor of staff	47
	being an evaluator	49
	aware of organisational change	53

3.   Management of the ward environment
        for:-   57
            the hospital as a whole   57
            the ward as a unit   58
            the ward visitor   61

4.   The acute ward as a learning environ-
        ment:-   65
            the student and meeting their
            competencies   68
            the organisation of the learning
            environment   90

Appendix I: Nursing, Midwifery and Health Visitors Rules
Approval Order 1989 No 1456   97

Index   99

Foreword

A newly qualified staff nurse was asked recently, *Do you normally have a high standard of organisation within your clinical area – or do you "just muddle along"?*' She paused. She thought. Her reply was very revealing.
'**We have a high standard of muddle!'**

This book will give those seeking to improve their organisational abilities an insight into the skills, knowledge and attitudes required to manage patient care effectively.

The format makes it 'user friendly', being concise, readable, coherent and appropriate to the changing needs of the late '90s'.

It also contains scenarios for group teaching and discussion. Although written as a book it could readily be utilised as distance learning material.

The needs of learners undertaking educational programmes are highlighted in the sections on the ward learning environment and guidance given to help manage student placements.

This book can be safely recommended to all those wishing to ably manage an acute ward.

Donna Winning
RGN, NDN, RCNT, Cert Ed

Acknowledgements

We would like to acknowledge the help of many people who have encouraged and supported us in the writing of this book.

Firstly thank you to the many colleagues and students we have met during our career and from whom we have learnt the needs of managers, both the fledgling and the experienced, especially in these times of change.

Our thanks go particularly to Donna Winning for kindly reading the various drafts and advising us, and to Sandra Fenwick for her help with the word processing...

Thanks also to Kath Butler for her special skills in compiling the illustrations for this book from a few tentative ideas.

Our especial thanks go to Dave and Mike for their support, encouragement and help during the compilation of this book.

Jane Walton
Maggie Reeves

Introduction

Nursing in the nineties is far removed from the secure world when the ward sister was mistress of all the ward she surveyed and the hierarchy was such that there were very clear lines of command and each member of the ward team had specific and prescribed tasks to perform.

There have been many changes in health care which have been fashioned by the social, political, cultural, economic and educational upheavals which have been the hallmark of the latter part of the twentieth century.

The implications of these changes have been felt very particularly in the ward areas. These have led to changed responsibilities of the staff of the wards, increased stress as these responsibilities have been absorbed (often with no preparation or training), and a need for greater adaptability from the nurses in the health care team.

How does a nurse manage the ward in the middle of the following demands? The hospital in which she works is seeking Trust status, the General Practitioners in the surrounding area are fund holders, the patients are more aware of their rights and the contents of the Patients' Charter (1992/1995). The ward for which she has responsibility will soon have a delegated budget at the same time as the patient turnover is faster and consequently the level of dependence of those on the ward is greater, and still the quality of the service nurses provide must be maintained at a high level.

In addition there is a reduction in the number of student nurses to supervise, and those who are allocated to the ward are supernumerary and different from the past. To keep abreast of the needs of the students, and personal professional needs, the nurse seeks to improve upon academic qualifications for which she may be given 50% financial support (but no time for college) at the same

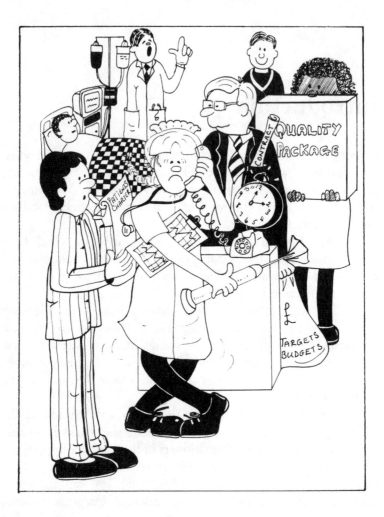

The Nurse

time as there is a contraction of services within the hospital and many of the staff face re-application for their jobs and the real possibility of redundancy. With such conflicts raging is there any wonder that morale is dropping and, with increased personal affluence, a job is harder to relinquish.

This book seeks to look at many of the pertinent situations any nurse may face, and the focus will be that of the acute care ward.

Each chapter seeks to address aspects of management.

The competencies relating to Project 2000 will be reviewed in the chapter on the learning environment as they are the requirements which have to be achieved by law before registration as a nurse can occur (see Appendix 1).

Although management theory will be referred to, the main aim of this book is to apply the principles of management to practice. It involves the reader in an assortment of exercises which will relate to themselves, their colleagues and their work place. Further reading is listed to expand the theoretical base.

This book does not intend to give all the answers, but to direct the reader to develop themselves.

It is directed at the established manager, the maturing manager and the fledgling manager.

1
Management of self and implications for the acute ward

This chapter looks at what a manager is.

The essence of management lies in the ability to achieve pre-determined goals through your own efforts and the efforts of other people with the most efficient and effective use of resources. A manager will have a function of completing many differing tasks.

They will need to be **motivated, skilled** and **competent.** Depending on how far away from the situation a manager is, the tasks of the manager may be different.

Essentially to complete the function or the tasks a manager needs to be competent as a :

Leader	**Controller**
Communicator	**Negotiator**
Planner	**Decision Maker**
Implementor	**Delegator**
	Motivator
Evaluator	

These skills indicate the various roles a manager has to perform and as such they will be discussed in more detail in subsequent sections of this book.

Each aspect will be looked at as it relates to:

1. The individual

2. The acute ward

3. Others.

Very often the roles on the list conflict and compete with others in the multi-disciplinary team. Further reading on role theories may be found in sociological studies.

One of the frustrations of management in the Health Service is the multiplicity of managers in all fields.

How does this affect you?

An exercise which might be useful to do at the outset is to create your own 'role map' to show what your role is in the organisation, and how these roles relate or conflict with your roles in another context.

Exercise

1.   *Take a large sheet of paper and draw a circle in the centre to represent yourself. Put your name and title in the circle.*

2.   *Divide the paper in half. The left hand side is your external role, eg. son/daughter, youth club leader, and the right hand side is your role in the organisation, eg. staff nurse E grade, union representative.*

3.   *Now make a 'spider gram' and draw the 'legs' of the spider at different lengths. Write at the end of the 'legs' the roles you play both in the organisation and out of it. The roles you perceive as more important put nearer to the 'body' of the 'spider' and further away as the role gets less important for you.*

4.   *On the relevant side of the page list the responsibilities the different roles place upon you. In addition try to think of the joys and pains that these roles bring you.*

5.   *Indicate on your role map which of the management expectations listed earlier are represented. Make a separate list of the expectations which are not.*

6.   *Compare your role map to your job description. Whether it*

matches or not, it will be a useful document to work from when you are next appraised.

7. *Do you have any areas of conflict or potential conflict between your organisational and external roles?*

This exercise may be pertinent as you consider the next section.

Management of self

The first person any manager, or aspiring manager, must manage is themselves. This will include the need to examine how they 'tick', how they manage their resources, such as time, what they value, how they lead and how they manage. Once there is an understanding of the self, then an examination of the role to be undertaken in the ward area will begin.

Time management

How do you manage your time ?

Much is written on time management but the following is a simple means of assessment and analysis.

Are you a careful planner, but so careful you get little done ?

Are you scatty and do things as they catch your eye ?

Are you slow and methodical but rather uninspiring ?

Are you a 'lists' person — writing lists to remind yourself to read other lists ?

Are you quick and intolerant of others, lamenting their inadequacies ?

Are you always, sometimes or never late ?

Are you bored easily, or can you while away a day and not bother where it has gone ?

*Are you the sort of person who always gets all the work
done, however much there is to do ?*

*Are you the busy person who is always given another
job to do because you always cope ?*

*Are you so bad at doing things that you are ignored in
favour of someone else?*

Whoever you are in this list, and maybe you are a combination of
several of the afore mentioned, an analysis of one's use of time is a
valuable exercise.

Any time-use exercise in nursing has a built-in ability to fail
because of the unexpected happenings likely to occur, particularly
on an acute ward. However, do not be daunted, use this simple
mnemonic L E A P S

L	list the activities to be done — in a day, in a week, on a shift, this can be done mentally or by literally writing a list
E	estimate the time needed for each activity
A	allow time for error / unscheduled activity
P	prioritise the activities — be ruthless
S	study the activities of the day

Consider:

Did you anticipate the majority of activities ?

Did you allow enough time ?

Were you side-tracked with non priority jobs, or by

ones you enjoyed doing but were not very important ?

Having completed this then:

Congratulate yourself on your successes

Plan to do better tomorrow

Evaluation of time can be done whilst travelling, having a bath or drinking a cup of coffee — it need not take long. If you insist on evaluating just as you are going off to sleep, we suggest you have pen and paper by your bed to jot things down.

On further reflection, perhaps every one should write things down to remove them from 'active thinking' to enable sleep to be uninterrupted.

This evaluation of time is the first step in determining how you function as a manager. It should also help you to gain / develop organisational and delegation skills.

Time is an expensive commodity and can be easily squandered in the nursing handover report, during meal breaks, and in trying to do things quickly, without thinking the action through. Whatever the pressure within the clinical environment, some management of time is pertinent and may well release you from self imposed pressures due to simple mismanagement, or gossiping.

Time management on the acute ward

Exercise

> *Apply the 'L E A P S' process to a recent day's activity on the ward or to a group of patients for whom you care.*

When managing one's time it is important to remember that everyone's time is valuable.

Time is probably your most valuable resource.

Time with regard to patient care on an acute ward can be looked at in two ways:

- *Indirectly*
- *Directly*

Indirect care *– it is possible that 50% of ward time is spent on activities* *that are not directly related to patient care.*

Consider the time taken in:

- *Answering the telephone*
- *Ordering supplies*
- *Collecting supplies*
- *Restocking*
- *Meetings*

Consider other activities that are indirect care.

Make a record of time spent on these activities and decide whether time is wasted here.

An aspect of indirect patient care that can affect the direct care dramatically is that of planning the off duty.

The planning of the off duty is a means of organising the ward so that the philosophy can be fulfilled, the nursing model applied and aspects such as appropriate level of material supplies maintained

Direct care — is patient care, and as such needs to be managed — it does not just 'happen'.

The manager must determine the patient needs in order to determine the staffing requirements to meet these needs. Taking account of the patient needs allows the nurse manager to:

- *Determine the number of staff that are required remembering to include meeting the named nurse expectation*
- *Determine when the staff are required*
- *Determine the skills mix of the required staff.*

In considering the patient's needs various factors need to be taken into account.

For example consider the time it takes to:

- *Bed-bath a patient as compared to an ambu-lift bath*
- *Feed a patient who is having swallowing difficulties*
- *Walk a patient to the toilet using a zimmer frame*
- *Give an injection.*

However do not forget that the acute care ward may change suddenly, this needs to be taken into account when considering patient needs.

Remember:

- *The possible admissions, especially if you are admitting directly from an accident and emergency department*
- *The change in patient needs due to investigations or operations*
- *The anticipated turnover of patients.*

When evaluating both the indirect and direct activities in the ward you should also consider the following:

- *Is the activity necessary?*
- *Is the most appropriate person completing the activity?*

Values clarification

The next step in self assessment is what do you value ? This links very well with time management. If you value the way you spend your time, then the above exercise may well have helped you conform with a value you wish to keep.

'Values Clarification' as a term was first discussed in the

1960s but the philosophers over the centuries have always discussed who and what we are by those things we value in life.

A value is:

> 'One of a set of personal beliefs and attitudes about the truth, beauty and worth of any thought, object or behaviour. They are action oriented and give direction and meaning to one's life.'
>
> (Simon 1973)

> 'If you do not take time to examine and articulate your values you will not be fully effective with patients.'
>
> (Uustal 1978)

In an ideal world something we value is:

- *Chosen*
- *Prized*
- *Acted upon.*

Our values are formed and influenced over the years by the following factors:

- personal
- political
- educational
- peers
- professional
- organisational
- national

- religious
- cultural
- family
- socio-economic
- media
- experiential

Whatever our values are, they will be challenged in nursing from the very first day on the ward until our retirement. Each person has 'values' and they are special to that individual and so can never be considered 'wrong' but may just be different from our own.

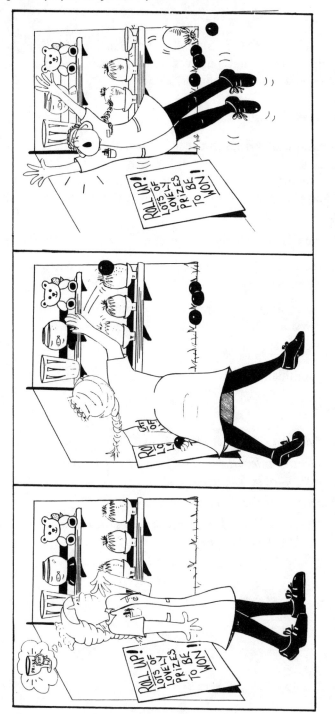

At the funfair I choose a particular game I prize selecting a prize to be won I act upon paying the money for a 'go' to win

Nevertheless, this can cause conflict when making decisions, when teaching patients and relatives, and are very pertinent when working in a multi-disciplinary team.

Implications of values in the acute ward

The following values may be particularly relevant to an acute ward and may be expressed by members of staff, patients and/or relatives.

1.   An individual's right to choose

2.   Human life is sacred and must not be terminated without a fight

3.   Psychological and spiritual care is more important than physical

4.   Personal security

5.   Confidentiality

Exercise

In the following sequence of scenarios

   Identify different values which are being expressed by each of the people involved.

   Decide the flash points which may occur.

   Consider which of the previous values each person might have to sacrifice ?

Scenarios.

You are working on an acute medical ward with 28 beds. Today is a typical busy morning and the staff whom you have allocated are as follows

| Staff Nurse A | } | 6 heavy patients requiring |
| 2nd Year student B | | the most care |

| Enrolled nurse C | } | 12 patients requiring some care |
| 3rd Year student | | |

| Nursing Care Assistant E | } | 10 patients requiring minimum |
| with some help from Yourself | | care |

A   By lunch time A and B have completed all their work. As usual, C and D have not finished their work and ask for help from A and B. This help is refused because they say that C has been disorganised and D has spent all morning chatting to the patients.

B   During the Senior Registrar's ward round that morning, Mr. Bracewell overhears that he has definitely got a malignancy. This is a possibility he has been asking from all the nurses for several days. His daughter has been adamant that Mr. Bracewell is not in a fit state to cope with the diagnosis.

C   Just before you go to lunch you hear from a Mrs. Green that a physiotherapist has asked her to attend a religious gathering when she is discharged from hospital. Mrs. Green asks if this is normal hospital policy and has she got something wrong with her that the hospital has not disclosed?

D   During the walk round report you are giving to the late shift, 76 year old Mrs. Smith, who has been told that a below knee amputation because of her very poor circulation and neuropathy is required, tells you that she was born with two legs and she will die with two legs ! You know Mrs. Smith's prognosis is very limited without the amputation.

E   Before you go off duty that afternoon the Directorate Nurse Manager informs you that due to sickness on the Coronary Care Unit, you will need to work there tomorrow. This is the one area in the hospital you have always dreaded.

This sequence scenario highlights some issues which you may have faced many times, rarely do we discover the correct answers, but we have to determine how we will react, behave and consequently support the other people involved in the situation.

Other values which are pertinent for each individual to consider are:

How do you demonstrate that you value your health ?

How do you demonstrate that you believe in individualised patient care?

Which age group do you prefer nursing and why ?

How should financial resources be allocated in clinical care?

Leadership

The next aspect of oneself which we will now examine is that of leadership and consequent managerial skills.

A manager must be a good leader.

If this is not the case then a leader emerges from the rest of the team. An inappropriate situation may then arise when, for example, a ward clerk or a nursing care assistant of long standing, becomes the actual leader.

Effective leadership is essential to good management. The designated leader does not just lead. Leadership involves managing demands made by others.

The manager must maintain leadership or delegate this role appropriately. It must also be remembered that for a leader to be effective there needs to be a team to carry out whatever needs to be done or, a 'followership'. (Heller & Van Til, 1982)

Leadership has been researched over the years and the results have fallen into the following categories:

What a leader is

What a leader does

What the situation demands.

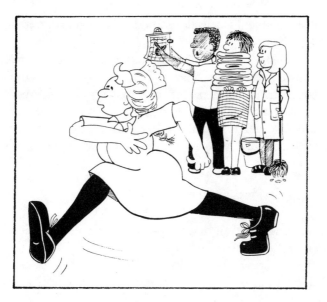

Sister will you 1..2..3..

What a leader is — trait theories

These theories are now considered to be rather outmoded however there seems to be an unwritten code in most organisations and this would include an acute ward. This code tends to reflect the findings of most of the 100+ studies in 'traits' that had taken place before 1950.

In a hospital context the unwritten code may include the following. A leader should be:

Knowledgeable/intelligent

Demonstrate initiative

Confident

Enthusiastic

Decisive

Approachable

A good communicator

Also it is possible that a leader should have an appropriate sense of humour.

This list could be endless depending on the type of ward, the team with which the leader works, and other individual characteristics which a person may have which enhances their leadership. This has been one of the criticisms of this group of theories. Another is that there have been leaders who could be termed successful, who were diffident, not very bright and indecisive.

What a leader does — behavioural theories

There is an assumption that people will work more efficiently and effectively if a certain style of leadership is employed or if the leader behaves in a certain way. Unfortunately some of the titles given to the leaders according to the style have a certain emotive aspect to them.

The styles can be seen along a continuum. At one end there is maximum leader control and minimum group freedom. At the other end there is maximum group freedom and minimum leader control. Please refer to Bernhard and Walsh (1990), p.59 in further reading list.

Thought also needs to be given to the style of leadership employed, such as authoritarian, democratic or permissive styles. In addition the day to day decisions will need consideration.

What the situation demands — contingency theories

The situation in an acute ward could demand many things from a leader. On a ward this changes from shift to shift and depends on the type of patients and what is happening to them. A normally democratic leader would need to be authoritarian in the following circumstances:

1.   Cardiac arrest

2.   New staff making up the majority of the work force

3.   Other emergency situations

4.   Disciplinary situations

Of the differing theorists perhaps the one which could be used most by nurses is John Adair(1983) who draws attention to:

- *The task*
- *The team*
- *The individual.*

so that each member of the team is suited to the overall task which needs to be performed.

As a ward leader/manager use the following exercise to consider the demands placed on you. Note that these demands link in with your management of time.

Exercise

> *What are your tasks today?*
>
> *Who is your team today?*
>
> *How many staff?*
>
> *What is the skill mix?*
>
> *What overlap exists with multi-disciplinary team?*
>
> *What special needs can be found in the individuals in your team? For example:*
>
> - *Time out for interview*
> - *Watching procedures*
> - *Dentist visit*
> - *Inexperience/ unqualified*
> - *Supernumerary status*
> - *Need for your mentorship.*

Consider whether your team is supported appropriately by outside agencies such as catering, cleaning and maintenance.

It may be pertinent after this barrage of questions to sit and think.

Reflect on the type of leader you are.

If you are not sure there are exercises to accompany the theories mentioned earlier which can give an indication of your preferred style.

There are several useful exercises regarding leadership in Isard (1987). The section on Improving Teamwork could be particularly useful.

This is an exercise which you could do to highlight some of the characteristics which you portray.

Consider the following list and underline seven characteristics which best describe you as a leader/manager.

ambitious	observant	assertive	practical
generous	independent	out-going	self-controlled
reliable	capable	conscientious	dependent
likeable	intellectual	dynamic	unpredictable
compromising	obedient	shy	moody
easily led	logical	thorough	self-disciplined
trustworthy	honest	perfectionist	lazy
indifferent	easily hurt	opinionated	disillusioned
argumentative	cautious	selfish	cynical
motivated	knowledgeable	adaptable	imaginative

Reflect on your answers and then consider if you think the characteristics listed are appropriate for management and whether there are areas which you could or should change.

Now show the list to a close friend or colleague whom you trust and ask whether or not they agree with your list. If they do not agree, take note of the differences and consider whether you demonstrate to others characteristics of which you are unaware.

This and other similar exercises can be quite harrowing if the results are not what you anticipate.

Having determined the type of leader you tend to be, this may need to be reviewed from time to time as your role within the organisation changes and develops. As a leader you must be prepared to lead and also to be consistent. If you put yourself in your followers footsteps, think how it must be if you are moody and inconsistent. You can't have a 'personality transplant' but you can curb excesses if you have them. Refer back to the characteristics list if you are not too sure if your behaviour could adversely affect the team.

Once you have decided on the type of person and or leader you are, it is now pertinent to consider the next aspect of management, the management of others.

References and further reading

Adair J (1983) *Effective Leadership*. Pan Books, London

Adair J (1985) *Effective Decision Making*. Pan Books, London

Adair J (1987) *Effective Team Building*. Pan Books, London

Bernhard L A & Walsh M (1990) *Leadership, the key to the professionalism of nursing*. 2nd Edn. C V Mosby, St Louis

Heller A Van Til (1982) cited in Koontz H (1988) *Management*. 9th Edn. Mc-Graw Hill, New York

Isard J (1987) Managing Care **Pack 4** *Improving Teamwork*. Distance Learning Centre, South Bank Polytechnic, London

Mersey Regional Health Authority (1991) Workload and skill mix management. *Using Information in Managing the Nursing Resource*. Greenhalgh and Company Ltd

Robbins S P (1973) *Essentials of Organisational Behaviour*. 3rd Edn. Prentice Hall International, London

Simon S B (1973) *Meeting yourself halfway* cited in Tschudin V (1992) *Values, a primer for Nurses*. Baillaire Tindall, London

Sullivan M P (1990) *Nursing Leadership and Management*. Spring House Corporation

Tschudin V (1993) Ethics: Nurses and Patients. Scutari Press, London

Uustal D (1978) Values Clarification in Nursing: Application to practice. *Am J Nurs*, **Dec** 2053-2063

VaughanB & Pillmoor M (Eds) (1989) *Managing Nursing Work*. Scutari Press, London

2
Management of others

This chapter will look at the management of others. There are some key skills, aspects of knowledge and pertinent attitudes which need to be fostered by any manager.

As an initial look at the management of others consider some of the skills, knowledge and attitudes related to the manager of a ward.

Compare the following identified skills with your roles listed at the beginning of chapter one.

Skills

- Communication
- Technical
- Teaching
- Delegation
- Negotiation
- Arbitration
- Observation
- Supervisory
- Listening
- Leadership
- Organisation
- Maintaining quality

Knowledge

- Law
- Policies
- Research
- Nursing competencies
- Ability
- Availability of all members of staff
- Procedures
- Job descriptions
- Professional issues
- Capability

Attitudes

- Fair
- Approachable
- Aware of own values

- Non-judgmental
- Self-controlled
- Aware of other's values

These skills, knowledge and attitudes should be channelled into your management role.

There are six elements of managerial leadership.

The manager /leader

1. Is competent as a professional nurse and as a leader

2. Leads by example

3. Is a good communicator

4. Ensures each member of the ward team is clear as to the ward's role and their individual role

5. Delegates appropriately upwards, downwards and sideways, and lets go once a task is delegated

6. Ensures all team members have the tools to do the job relating to the environment, equipment and training

Some of these elements of a manager's role will now be looked at in detail.

Being competent

The awarding of the registered nurse qualification is based on successful achievement of the competencies as stated in Rule 18A, The Nurses Rules. (See Appendix 1)

The Code of Professional Conduct (1992) states that a registered nurse is personally accountable for their practice.

At this juncture it is vital to discuss the notions of responsibility and accountability. Management when undertaken by a third year student nurse will carry a different level of accountability from the 'G' grade.

Responsibility is a charge for which one is answerable. Patient care could be classed as a responsibility.

Accountability is explaining, defining or measuring in some way the results of decision making.

Accountability cannot be expected from everyone. It can only be attained once knowledge, ability and responsibility have been achieved and authority has been given. This can be likened to a ladder. Each rung has to be climbed before accountability can be expected.

Rung 5. Accountability

This need to justify one's acts of omission and commission is clearly documented in the UKCC's Exercising Accountability(1989), and Standards for the Administration of Medicines(1992) booklets. It is something as citizens which we take on without much thought as we mature into adults. As nurses it is something we are prepared for and we develop into, but none-the-less it needs to be considered and treated with respect.

Rung 4. Autonomy

This much discussed topic is necessary if true accountability is demanded. Most nurses are only nominally autonomous as there are many others who make up the multi-disciplinary team whose position must be accommodated thus diluting autonomy.

Rung 3. Authority

Authority is a status which is conferred in different ways. It can be ascribed or earned. In nursing, authority is normally conferred and is closely linked to knowledge and ability and lately to job description and grading.

Rung 2. Responsibility

Throughout this time, responsibility will be given to the nurse. Charges will need to be fulfilled and tasks completed. The nurse will be responsible for carrying out these tasks, and the quality of these tasks. The more senior the nurse becomes, the type of task will change and the level of responsibility.

Rung 1. Ability

A nurses ability in the areas of skills knowledge and attitudes is developed during her pre-registration education. Whether a foundation course or common foundation programme is followed there will be a minimum level expected of every registered nurse. Once qualified the nurse will still be learning and developing in line with Post Registration Education Practice (PREP) and The Scope of Professional Practice (UKCC1992). Different abilities will be developed building on the pre-registration programme.

Adapted from Bergman (1981)

With all the current changes in the National Health Service(NHS) how much of this affects the levels of nurses responsibilities?

Organisational structure has changed to accommodate other hierarchical structures within the health service. The development of ward clerk's roles and the separate hierarchical structure and functioning of domestic staff have altered the lines of responsibility and communication. The reduction of junior doctors hours also has implications for nurses accountability. Will financial consideration mean the discontinuation of some services and the redefinition of nursing responsibilities?

It is of importance to note here that within The Code of Professional Conduct (1992) it states,

> *'ensure that no action or omission on your part, or within your sphere of responsibility, is detrimental to the interests, condition or safety of patients and clients.'*

Does this mean that the ward manager is ultimately responsible for the state of the ward environment? The role has for some time now been undertaken by domestic staff who have their own formal hierarchical structure. However, is it the ultimate responsibility of the ward manager? This area is still very unclear.

Within change of responsibility there will also be aspects such as delegating appropriately.

It may be helpful at this point to refer to the role map exercise from the first chapter.

Consider to whom and for what you are accountable in the two arenas, one as a citizen and the other as a nurse, and fill in any gaps with your own areas of accountability.

For example

1. As a citizen you are accountable

To	For
• Bank for loan	• Mortgage
• Local Council for Council Tax	• Pets
• To law when driving	• Children's schooling

2. As a nurse you are accountable

To	For
• UKCC	• Drug administration
• Your employer	• Student supervision
• Own manager	• Patient care

Within an organisation it is important to note the rules and regulations which affect you as they may constitute the charge for which you are answerable.

The regulations may be from health and safety, professional or organisational discipline or laws. The NHS being a bureaucratic organisation has many of its own regulations also.

Exercise: Make a chart of the laws, rules and regulations which affect your working environment.

This may be an exercise the ward team can develop together so that the supporting documents can be available to consult.

Consider the rules and regulations by which the ward is managed, and consider the source of their origin and the consequences of non-adherence.

Sources of rules and regulations in the ward environment

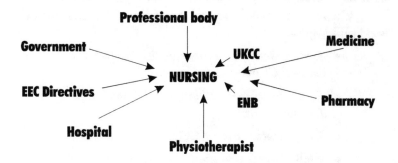

Rules and Regulations

As can be seen some rules and regulations have arisen from managers at governmental level whereas others have arisen from local hospital level. The professional bodies have also stated their requirements.

Chart of examples of documentation of rules and regulations

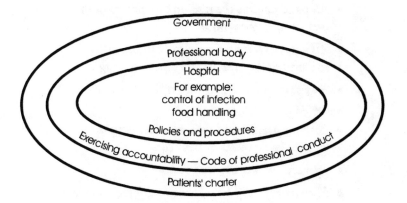

A means of linking the 'rules' and 'regulations' to practice on the ward may be disciplinary action due to non-adherence, or could be a written statement of intent as found in the ward philosophy.

The philosophy forms the ward outcome and should link with the overall outcome of the health care organisation.

Consider the following and determine their link with the ward philosophy:

- *Government documentation, for example, the Patients Charter named nurse*
- *Statements found within local Hospital Trust documentation*
- *Competencies and UKCC advisory booklets*
- *ENB/ Higher education expectations*
- *Hospital procedures/ contracts.*

Each area will vary but an example of a philosophy is shown below. This needs to be drawn up in agreement with the ward team and made available for all to see.

Other documents will complement the philosophy, these include policies, procedures and standard setting statements.

The philosophy

- *All patients have the right to care provided by a suitably qualified nurse*
- *All patients have the right to be informed concerning the care that they are receiving*
- *Any patient has the right to refuse care without fear of prejudice*
- *Both the patient and their relatives have the right to be involved in their care*
- *Privacy and dignity will be honoured*
- *Each patient will be informed with regard to the nurse or nurses that are responsible for their care*
- *Confidentiality will be maintained*

- *Each member of the ward team is recognised for the part that they contribute to the ward care*
- *There is a recognised need for staff support within the ward team to the mutual benefit of all*
- *Nursing theory and research will be incorporated into care to improve the quality of patient care and staff morale.*

Being competent both as a nurse and a manager will allow you to perform your managerial role and control the ward situation.

Controller

Control, whether it is self applied or otherwise, is not always appreciated by some but may be second nature to others. A manager must have some degree of control over activities. An individual manager may find their control ratio is dependent on their leadership style.

A controller needs someone or something to control. An active and a passive element.

As a ward manager you should have some form of control over the staff on the ward.

Exercise

Make a list of all the staff on the ward and consider whether you have the ultimate control. Look at the medical, domestic and secretarial staff as well as the nursing staff.

In completing this exercise you may become aware that the managers control is based on an hierarchical structure, that is the manager controls grades below their own, be it grade D, E, F, or G. Control related to other disciplines is managed through their hierarchical structure.

Control, however, needs to be communicated, (see section on communication).

Remember some good must come out of the control. For example:

- *The best record in pressure sore prevention*
- *The only ward with an underspend.*

The ward controller can be the agent for the hospital or health trust to ensure the correct policies and procedures are carried out, as discussed in the last section.

Control is now being incorporated into the ward manager's role with respect to budget holding and maintenance of quality.

Control, to be effective, has to be a motivating force for the ward team. If it is a means of 'punishment' it will be resented and only complied with reluctantly.

It is not always possible to ensure that control is kept.

Communicator

Much has been written on this subject and yet it is an area within nursing that gets forgotten.

Communication within any organisation may be formal or informal. Much communication goes on through informal channels in social contact and can give rise to rumour. The coffee time gossip that starts with, "Have you heard", or "Tell me the latest".

Informal lines can give rise to anxiety and exaggeration.

Imagine the effect of the following statement, '60% of staff are going to be made redundant!'.

Within the organisation communication should follow formal rules.

Adherence to formal lines of communication can prevent misunderstanding or unnecessary anxiety.

From a manager's point of view it is important to acknowledge that lines of communication are along lines of authority, or should be. Although access is granted to higher levels in the organisational structure communication should go formally through each level in turn.

Exercise

On a piece of paper draw a circle which represents your ward, then

1.   Outline the hierarchical structure of managers within health
        care in your organisation, you should end with the Secretary
        of State.

2.   List the areas or units that link to your area from the hospital
        environment, draw them in relationship to your ward with
        the most important nearest to the ward circle.

3.   List the various personnel that link with your area and then
        draw them also in relationship to your ward.

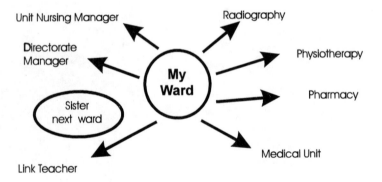

**An example of the areas and some of the personnel that may
link to your ward**

Not only is it important to recognise lines of communication but it is also important to know how and when people in the structure can be communicated with at any time, remembering that not all of them will have a bleep system arrangement. This will mean that you have to have a full understanding of the need and means to contact these people, in other words you will need to understand their role and responsibilities along with the lines of communication.

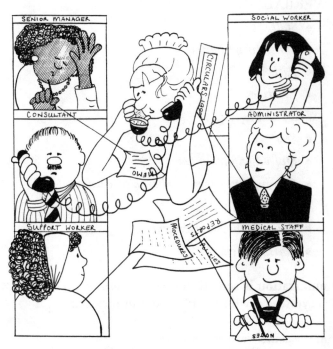

Who should you speak to!

Communication between nurses and doctors crosses hierarchical, bureaucratic links and is related to their role.

Consider the situation when the ward manager questions a drug prescription that a junior doctor has ordered. Does the manager speak to the junior doctor or the house officer or the consultant or does the manager take the query to the junior or senior pharmacist? Who will tell the junior doctor that they cannot prescribe the amount of drug that they have?

Organisations work within rules and regulations so that the answers to many of these situations can be found in documentation. For example if a drug is not prescribed correctly the rules and regulations can be shown to the doctor.

Key areas to consider for communication:

VERBAL

- *Staff*
- *Multi-disciplinary team*
- *Patients*
- *Relatives*

WRITTEN

- *Staff*
- *Multi-disciplinary team*
- *Community / primary health care team*
- *Hierarchy*
- *Educational establishments*
- *Nursing press*

Communication is something we all think we do rather well. It's everyone else who is bad at communicating.

Within the acute ward remember:

> *Give others the courtesy you would expect yourself. It is difficult when you are busy to maintain consistency*

> *Do not use a different voice or persona when you are talking to the domestic and when you are talking to the consultant*

> *Written communication is one area in which nurses generally perform badly.*

Communication is an area of quality which costs nothing but thought.

Communication should be:

- *Accurate*
- *On time*
- *Given to the appropriate person*
- *Clear*
- *Concise*
- *Coherent*

Communication will allow you as a manager to negotiate, motivate, plan and delegate.

Refer to, the UKCC booklet (1993) *Standards for Records and Record Keeping, 4–6.*

Negotiator

This is a term which seems to fit better with the sales department or in industry rather than nursing. However, much negotiating takes place on every ward, every day.

Consider the last week and identify situations in which you have 'negotiated'.

Whatever happens during negotiation, both parties involved want (or should want) to reach a mutually acceptable conclusion. Ideally, each party should be prepared to move from its original position, otherwise one party has an unfair advantage.

Look back at the list you prepared. Do you consider a mutually acceptable conclusion was reached on every occasion?

How far from your original position did you move?

Nurses have long tried to negotiate with patients over their care. In the present climate the negotiation is for different commodities. Negotiations for finance, staff, contracts and students are on many agendas. Negotiating is like bartering in a bazaar.

Here are 10 golden rules for negotiating:

1. Know how much you have to spend

2. Start off by asking for more than you can get

3. Listen hard whilst the opponent speaks

4. Challenge position – are they bluffing ?

5. Concessions should be conditional. I will...if you will...

6. Speak firmly and assertively, but do not make your opponent look foolish

7. Look for ways of maintaining the dignity of all parties

8. Clarify the position when it is considered finalised

9. Make your decision clear to your opponent

10. Remember that most negotiating within the health service can have a 'knock on' effect for patient care

If it is possible, watch someone else negotiate before you get involved. You can learn by someone else's positive or negative experience.

Consider the negotiations that may go on in deciding how to meet the patient's needs. For example for discharge or self medication. Patient care should be negotiated with the patient in a patient centred manner wherever possible, but you should also consider what the hospital rules and regulations say about the situation.

Consider the situation when as a manager you may have to negotiate for more staff. You may wish to read further on assertiveness at this point, but remember you should have a justified reason for your negotiation. Justified reason requires evidence of a factual nature, so collect your facts but do not forget to use rules and regulations, or research evidence to support your negotiation.

In all aspects of management it is important to **plan** your strategy, as an aspect of the problem solving process, (see also decision making section).

Planner

When planning it is important to determine:

1. Who is responsible

2. Who will convert the plan into goals

3. Who will put the plans into action

4. Who will check progress

5. Who will evaluate

Planning the management of time as an example should overspill into the whole ward. There are many occasions when communally the ward team waste their time.

As a useful activity (and assessment of your situation) list some of the actual or potential areas of time wasting on your ward.

Potential time wasting situations are asked for as it is worth trying to tighten up on these, particularly if you are in the situation of battling for more resources. You cannot be seen to be wasting the resources you already have.

Within your list there may be the following situations given as examples which cry out for better management on many wards.

Potential Problem	Possible Solution
1. 'Chatty' handover reports or duplication/triplication of handover	Self discipline time limit
	Consider style of handover. Should more information be included in care plan?
	Should all the ward team be involved in handover? Could teaching be done at another time?
	Communicate verbally then put it in writing after changes occur, eg after ward rounds.
2 Meal breaks - staff taking too long	Start breaks early so staff are not too tired. State break times in advance so there are no hold-ups waiting for someone to be ready to go on time. Do not send too many staff at once - experiment with 2 at a time.
	Remember your skill mix.
3. Unbalanced off-duty rotas	It is hard to refuse requests for off-duty but the good of the ward must take precedence over the individual.
	Try different patterns of off-duty until you find one which suits your area, eg a fixed shift pattern per week.
	Try putting internal rotation of nights so that a member of staff does a block of nights rather than 'chopping and changing'.
	Remember your skill mix.

Potential Problem	Possible Solution
4. Patients/Relatives Unplanned chats regarding discharge, preparation for treatment.	Book time to talk to patients and relatives so that time is not wasted later.
5. One-off teaching/patient education sessions.	Are there several patients who would benefit from a chat on a certain subject? This may help with patients giving each other support. Questions may also be asked by one patient which another may not have thought of.
6. Multi-disciplinary team	Determine which 'rounds' are essential for nursing staff to attend. Communicate with relevant personnel, so that if a nurse is not present on the round, there is a good communication network.

A way around some of these problems could be through advanced planning and could be incorporated into the off-duty planning. This should enable you to programme teaching sessions, doctors rounds, mentor supervision, theatre days, admission days and other recurring ward activities so that on paper at least you can demonstrate that you have utilised your personnel to the best of your ability.

Remember to consider patient dependencies and who can manage and who can implement care.

Completing the duty rotas is difficult and time consuming, it is advisable to arrange a quiet undisturbed time to complete this.

Remember you cannot do everything; teaching sessions and doctors rounds, to name but two. Prioritise and decide what you can do. Then divide that into **must, should, could** do, tasks.

Planning the off-duty need not be a sole responsibility of the manager but may be delegated appropriately. However the manager must remember who is ultimately accountable and ensure that the rota is correct. The duty rota needs to consider various factors but it should be a balance between patient and staff requirements with the balance to the patients benefit.

Duty rotas therefore require the consideration of the skills mix of staff.

As a manager you should know your staff

This will include a knowledge of a number of permanent members of staff but also a number of transient staff, which could include students from any number of courses, some of which may be pre or post-registration and nursing staff from an agency or bank which may range from auxiliary to registered nurse.

How to know your staff

It may not be all that long before the nurse manager is able to interview and select and determine the working contracts of the ward team. At present, the G grade manager is responsible for the work produced by the members of the team whether it is delegated or not.

Therefore it is important that the manager has a good record of the staff job specifications and their capabilities. This is not as a rule a documented record kept by the ward manager but it is kept by the nursing officer or equivalent.

The ward manager may also be in the position of terminating the contract of a member of the ward team. It is therefore suggested that a record is maintained. This record may prove invaluable when wards are audited and when the requirements of PREP are taken into account. The acquisition of extended role capabilities will need to be taken into account when deciding job responsibilities, skill mix and staffing levels, all of which are essential considerations in the organisation of the staffing on the ward.

A point to consider is that the maintenance of the staff record need not be the sole responsibility of the ward manager but could be maintained by the staff members themselves. However it needs to be kept in a place that is easily accessible to both the manager and the members of staff.

Remember that staff should be keeping their own record as well, in the form of a profile. For information on profiling see further reading section.

The profile could serve as the ward record but will also be utilised when the nurse is required to re-register or on application for a new post.

An example of a suggested ward record.

Staff Record

Name _____

  Commencement of employment _____

Qualifications

  Management courses attended _____

  Teaching course attended _____

  Mentor/assessor/supervisor status _____

  Extended practice record _____

Any courses being currently undertaken:

  Course title _____

  Expected qualification _____

  Date of completion _____

  Particular needs to fulfil PREP _____

  Special strengths/interests eg wound care _____

  Date of re-registration _____

  Date of last appraisal _____

  Date of next appraisal _____

The staff record must meet the requirements of the job description. However there may be some unclear areas. Look at the following exercise.

Exercise

Identify areas of role/skill conflict which exist on your ward

- *Your own role*
- *Trained nursing staff*
- *Support staff.*

Analyse why these conflicts have arisen and suggest possible solutions.

You may need to consider the decision making process and then look at the appropriateness of delegation, (see later sections).

Nurses are very used to the nursing process and need to relate this problem solving cycle to aspects of ward life. In planning it is also important that the management strategy of the ward is recognised and considered.

The ward management strategy

Exercise

In order to consider your overall function as a ward manager review the following:

- *How is patient care managed?*
- *How is the named nurse requirement accommodated?*
- *What is the underlying nursing theory?*

Management of patient care

There are several methods of management including team nursing and primary nursing.

Team nursing must include a leader or organiser, this need not necessarily be the qualified nurse, but there must be a qualified nurse within the team to ensure that correct care is being carried out.

Primary nursing may be viewed as being in line with the named nurse approach, in that the patient is given a particular nurse to assess and plan their care. This will mean that the first level nurse must also have an 'associate nurse/s' who can carry out the care when they are not available. Primary nursing, means that the patients need to be arranged between the first level nurses. In either team nursing or primary nursing the nurse may be responsible for the patients who are:

- *On one side of the ward*
- *In a bay*
- *A range of high and low dependency patients from various areas of the ward.*

Whichever method is decided on it must be suitable to the:

- *Ward layout*
- *Patients' needs.*

Implications of ward layout on the management of patient care

The Nightingale ward. This ward invariably has patients who are more highly dependent in an area of easy access and visibility. To enable an even division of workload the staff are often allocated patients from both high and low dependency. Therefore it is often the case of dividing the ward into two with one team of nurses taking the left side and the other taking the right.

The Bay ward. The high dependency patients in this ward are often nearer the nurses station, visibility from the nurses station is good but not from other areas of the ward. Team nursing in this situation often means that the nurses take all or some patients in a bay and their patient allocation is spread throughout the ward. This creates problems with availability and visibility of the nurse both for the patient and the nurse.

Meeting the need of the named nurse requirement

The manager should ensure that each patient is aware of the nurse that is responsible for their care. As the manager you should ensure that

- *Nursing staff are aware of their responsibilities with regard to their patients*
- *The nurse has the appropriate qualifications to care for that patient*
- *The nurse will be available during that patients care or the nurse is replaced as soon as possible*
- *The nurse knows to refer problems appropriately.*

Remember that the management of care using a primary nurse is in line with the named nurse concept but do ensure that the relationship between the patient and the nurse is working to their mutual benefit.

The underlying nursing theory will affect the approach to nursing care.

It has been well recognised that the overall approach to nursing care follows the stages dictated by the nursing process. Assessment is the first stage followed by planning, implementation and finally evaluation. The philosophy of the area usually will have identified that its prime objective is to ensure safe patient care. This is often undertaken within the stages of the nursing process.

As the manager of the acute area it is necessary to know **who** is able to carry out each of the stages of the nursing process, **who** can supervise and **who** must be supervised in the implementation of care.

Within the format of the nursing process a variety of nursing models may be utilised. The models may be used on all patients or selectively, they may be used in their entirety or segmentally in combination with other models.

Each nursing model is said to consist of 4 or 5 factors referred to as parameters:

View of a person

View of the environment

View of health and/or illness

View of the nurse

View of nursing

The selection of the model of care within your ward may be dictated by the documentation that you are required to use and so this may be where your considerations need to start.

- *Do you have a set admission form/ care plans?*
- *Where have the forms originated from?*
- *Is it a requirement to use these forms only?*
- *What would be the procedure of change?*

The form needs to be examined to determine its link with a nursing model. It may be that your considerations need to include other ward areas due to patient transfer, eg. admission wards.

Review the structure of nursing models and decide the strategy of the ward.

A well planned ward management strategy should be in line with the ward philosophy, (see page 26).

Decision maker

Inherent in every facet of the role of a manager is the need to make decisions.

The nursing process is a problem solving cycle. The decision making cycle is similar but more extensive.

Oldcorn (1982) suggests that there are 6 stages:

1. **Identify/recognise the problem**
    Decide

    Is it my problem? ⟶ Is it someone else's problem?

    deal with it ↓ ignore it or offer help

    speculate if it will become your problem

2. **Diagnose the cause**
    Look for the cause – not symptoms
    Determine the facts – do not make an **assumption**
    As when you assume – Make an **ass** of **you** and **me**

3. **Identify possible solutions**
    Think in the plural and use all means and personnel at your disposal

4. **Evaluate the possible**
    Consider the pros and cons of the workable solutions

5. **Choose the solution**
    This can take courage when the decision has to be made during a time of general upheaval and uncertainty

6. **Implement the decision**
    In addition you will need to judge the effectiveness of your action

These six stages are sometimes portrayed as a cycle as we are always having to make decisions, many of which are on-going.

However beware of timing.

Choose the person to act out the decision if it is not going to be you. If it is to be someone else, check the delegation list first, (see page 46).

Delegator

Delegation is an activity that is sometimes accompanied by a sense of guilt and failure. There are at least two ways of considering the art of delegation.

An, *'I can't cope with my workload and so I'm offloading it on to you'* type of syndrome.

This occurs particularly when management skills are first being developed. However, another way of looking at delegation is seeing it as according someone else the dignity of this task or responsibility.

The person to whom the task or responsibility has been delegated could see it as, *'more work for me – they never manage properly'* or that the delegation is a compliment in that they are deemed capable.

Inconsistent delegation is something to avoid. One day, when it suits you, give a person a task which they enjoy and succeed in doing. The next day, and with no explanation, you either do the task yourself or give it to a third person. This both breeds resentment and fosters lack of confidence in your colleagues.

Another pitfall of delegation is that it is easy to lack assertiveness when delegating. You feel you are grovelling to the delegate. This does nothing for your self respect and confidence. Use the authority which goes with your managerial position, but remember that it does not cost anything to say *'please'*.

No one person is indispensable. This is hard to take when you are submerged under your work.

The following are 8 stages to delegation. These can be applied upwards, downwards and sideways.

1.   Decide what must be delegated

2.   Decide the delegate – ensure they are competent/appropriate/accountable

3.   Determine willingness of delegate

4.   Communicate clearly and specifically to delegate. If necessary identify resources

5.   Allow the delegate to perform the activity

6.   Make provision for feedback/de-briefing if necessary

7.   Was the delegate successful?

8.   You are both successful if the results are successful

Always check with Code of Professional Conduct (UKCC 1992) and Exercising Accountability (UKCC 1989) and Scope of Professional Practice (UKCC 1992) to make sure you have delegated appropriately.

Implementor

Nurses are good 'doers', but not always so good at thinking first and assessing the situation and planning what to do. The most often seen situation is that of a wound dressing. How many times have you started the procedure only to find you have omitted one vital item from the proceedings?

The other aspect of implementation that needs to be considered when in management is how much of the nursing work should you do?

Don't let your guilt overtake the need for you to do different, but just as important 'management' work. This is not a carte blanche excuse to sit in the office all day and drink coffee !

- *Plan*
- *Decide*
- *Delegate*
- *And negotiate if necessary.*

But also remember you may need to *motivate* not only yourself but your staff.

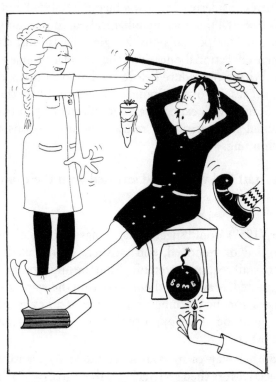

There are many theories of motivation

Motivator

A manager often has to motivate those who are being managed. This can also include self motivation. We all have those days...those weeks...those months...depending on our mood or environment.

There have been a variety of theories from Maslow (1954), with his hierarchy of needs through Hertzberg's(1959) motivation-hygiene theory and management by objectives (M.B.O.) to name but three. One aspect with which all theorists would concur is that motivation is necessary, either internal or external. The force that motivates and the effectiveness of motivation are two of the factors which are disputed.

When considering Maslow's hierarchy (1954) and the ward team, it is essential that each member feels an important individual in the group. That person's physiological needs must also be met before their educational ones. To send a student nurse to observe a long and tiring procedure before she has even had a drink that morning because of oversleeping, does not motivate that student to learn. Similarly to expect high commitment from trained staff when annual leave has been refused for no obvious reason, is wishful thinking.

How can staff feel valued and satisfied with their day's work?

Hertzberg(1959) would suggest that things that dissatisfy the staff, be controlled or removed, and satisfiers be installed. Maybe a member of staff requires 'stretching' and the opportunity to pursue study is granted. Maybe another role within the ward team such as co-ordinator for the teaching programme or a key worker in the lifting programme or the opportunity to do some research would motivate others.

Another way of motivating could be by identifying ward goals, objectives are then set to achieve these goals and achievement and performance is subsequently appraised or evaluated.

Job achievement or job satisfaction.

Each member of an organisation has a part to play otherwise they would not be employed. However we all need motivation to achieve and this motivation often comes from the manager.

Aspects to consider in motivating staff

Recognise them

- as an individual
- as a holder of a role
- as members of staff who have particular interests which they have developed, such as wound care, stoma care, pressure area care
- for their potential development

- remember their name!
- for their special skills
- for their own needs. This may relate to the planning of off-duty or to their educational needs

Continual, repetitive work may lead to decreased motivation and production, a change or a challenge within the remit of their job description may provide a stimulus to motivate the person.

Consider whether there is a project or a task group that may be appropriate for a member of staff to join but be careful not to overload the member of staff.

Beware you do not, *'flog a willing horse'*.

Following recognition, utilise their skills appropriately and, more importantly, acknowledge their contribution.

Recognition of staff may arise from assessment but may be identified on evaluation especially through the staff appraisal.

Evaluator

To evaluate there needs to be a standard or goal against which to measure your activity. How else can you say you have achieved something ? The old adage *'if you aim at nothing you hit it'* is pertinent here. Nurses seem to find goal setting quite difficult. To be of value a goal needs to be SMART.

- *S pecific*
- *M easurable*
- *A chievable*
- *R ealistic*
- *T ime related*

(Health Pick-Up 1994)

Not only does a manager need to ensure that goals are set for patient care, but the standards which are being set in many hospitals relating to the Patients' Charter (1992) also need to be achieved. These often include standards for reception onto the ward. Waiting time for the telephone to be answered. Method of approach by staff to patients and many, many more. The more workable your standards and goals are, the greater effect they will have on the atmosphere of your ward and also on your ability to evaluate them. These may be implemented on your ward already.

Exercise

Identify any evaluation tools that you may be using to measure patient care attainment or resource needs and outline their constraints.

The tools could include any that evaluate the following:

- *Staff appraisal*
- *Educational audit*
- *Patient goal achievement*
- *Patient satisfaction.*

Staff appraisal is viewed as a two way process.

The staff member has an opportunity to discuss how their job is progressing and to discuss their future progress. The manager can discuss the staff members progress and support or advise on future progress.

Consider:

- *When were you last appraised?*
- *What does your organisation require in the way of appraisal?*

Educational audit

A two way process when the ward can see and discuss the learning opportunities on the ward and the ward manager can discuss the learning needs of the educational establishment. Various theoretical, academic and practical aspects will be discussed which means that the ward staff should be prepared for an audit by considering the following:

- *What is the ward philosophy?*
- *What is the underlying model of nursing that facilitates the care?*
- *What type of patients does the ward have?*
- *How is the nursing documentation completed?*
- *How are the staff prepared for the role of teaching?*
- *What programme of teaching is available on your ward?*

Each educational establishment will have an audit document which is completed at the time of the audit so ask for a copy prior to the audit and also request a copy of the completed document. Your link teacher may well be the person to consult.

Patient goal achievement

Measuring patient care is not an easy task but there are some tools that can be used:

- *Observations*
- *Patient comments*
- *Research data.*

Whichever tool is used it relies on the fact that the goal has been set appropriately but it must also recognise the fact that conditions change and the pre-set goal may not be obtainable for a number of reasons and it must then be changed.

Goal-setting is a continuous process.

A few guidelines, ask yourself:

- *Is the goal realistic?*
- *Is it measurable?*
- *Is there an appropriate measuring tool?*

Patient satisfaction

It is the nurses aim to provide quality care for the patient but the patient and their carers must, wherever possible, be involved in the decisions regarding their care and they must be given the opportunity to discuss the attainment of their care needs. This may be measured in some wards by the receipt of letters or cards of thanks for the care given both from the patient or the relative, or by the letters of complaint. These are not the only methods of evaluation of patients satisfaction.

Like all methods of evaluation it must go on over a period of time so ask your patients on a frequent basis and remember that the patient who might state his/her dissatisfaction is only providing you with the information you need to evaluate your ward. They are not the patient to ignore, or label as the unpopular patient, but the patient to listen to and diagnose the cause of dissatisfaction and act on it. There are also documented tools that may be used to measure patient care and satisfaction.

Following evaluation change may be necessary.

The organisational structure and change

The NHS as an organisation is subject to constant change.

This change can be:

- *Endogenous – from within*
- *Exogenous – from without (enforced).*

Whichever route the change travels on, the organisation can be used effectively to outline a strategy to deal with change.

Utilising the information with regard to organisational structure and function (see further reading section), it is possible to outline a strategy to deal with change.

1. Identify the type of managerial control. This will allow you to know:
   - *Who will make the decisions*
   - *The lines of communication*

2. Ensure the intended outcomes are clearly set with time limits where possible. Ensure that these time limits are attainable.

3. Involve the appropriate personnel either on a full-time basis or within reasonable work expectations. Consider whether a project or a task force would be suitable.

4. Communicate through formal lines frequently but appropriately.

5. Accept and respect the contribution of the staff.

6. Encourage and manage appropriately.

Finally consider whether:

- *Your ward organisation is bureaucratic or hierarchical*
- *Staff and patients views are taken into account in decision making*
- *Power and control are all yours or are delegated to you*
- *All your staff are aware of their roles*
- *The ward management strategy and outcomes are known.*

References and further reading

Bergman R (1981) Accountability - Definition and Dimensions. *Intl Nurs Rev* **28**(2), pp 53-59

Brown R A (1992) *Portfolio Development and Profiling for Nurses.* Tingle J (Ed). 2nd Edn. Quay Books, Mark Allen Publishing Ltd, Dinton, Salisbury

Chinn P L & Kramer M K (1991) *Theory and Nursing, a systematic approach.* 3rd Edn. Mosby Year Book, St Louis

Department of Health (1993) *Health of the Nation, targeting practice contributions of nurses, midwives and health visitors.* Department of Health, London

Hertzberg F (1959) *The Motivation to work.* J Wiley & Sons, New York

Hunt J W (1992) *Managing people at work.* 3rd Edn. McGraw-Hill Book Company, London

Hyett K (1988) *Nursing Management Handbook.* Churchill Livingstone, Edinburgh

Marriner-Tomey A (1988) *Guide to Nursing Management.* 4th Edn. Mosby Year Book, St Louis

Marriner-Tomey A (1989) *Nursing Theorists and their work.* 2nd Edn. C V Mosby Company, Baltimore

Marson S, Hartlebury M, Johnston R, Scammell B (1990) *Managing People.* Macmillan, London

Mersey Regional Health Authority (1991) Workload and skill mix management. *Using Information in Managing the Nursing Resource*. Greenhalgh and Company Limited

NHS Training Directorate (1994) *Health Pickup. Management skills for health care professionals*. NHS

Oldcorn R (1982) *Management: A fresh approach*. Pan Books, London

Department of Health (1992) *Patients' Charter*. Department of Health, London

Department of Health (1995) *Patients' Charter & You*. Department of Health, London

Robbins S P (1992) *Essentials of Organisational Behaviour*. (3rd Edn). Prentice Hall International, London

UKCC (1987) *Confidentiality*. UKCC, London

UKCC (1989) *Exercising Accountability*. UKCC, London

UKCC (1992) *The Scope of Professional Practice*. UKCC, London

UKCC (1992) *Code of Professional Conduct.* UKCC, London

UKCC (1992) *Standards for the Administration of Medicines*. UKCC, London

UKCC (1993) *Standards for Records and Record Keeping*. UKCC, London

Vaughan B & Pillmoor M (Eds) (1989) *Managing Nursing Work*. Scutari Press, London

3
Management of the ward environment

It is now intended to look at the immediate work environment of the hospital and the ward and consider how these structures affect management.

Hospital environment

Florence Nightingale's philosophy featured the environment as a very prominent issue. Is this something we have grown complacent about as traditional domestic tasks no longer appear to be a nursing responsibility? The environment however is influenced by more than the domestic tasks.

Consider the expectations and considerations of your hospital:

- *Is it welcoming? Remember that many people come to hospital anxious and distressed. Does there appear to be a concerned welcome?*

- *Is it informative? How are people informed with regard to location and direction within the hospital?*

- *Is it safe? Is the environment well maintained and are hazardous material controlled appropriately?*

Hospitals can be strange and bewildering places not only for patients but for their relatives as well as nursing staff who may be new to the area or new to the job. Remember your first days – whether you are reading this book as a newly qualified nurse manager or as an experienced manager who may have recently changed your work environment.

It is important to know the lay-out of your hospital and where available offices, services and stores are located.

It is also important to have available the opening times of the services that may be required by the ward such as the stores department or pharmacy.

This information may be available in your ward but

- *Is it easily available?*

- *Is it kept in separate places?*

- *Has it been kept up-dated?*

Changes within the hospital environment are meaning that some services are being moved, closed down or expanded or that there is a change in their availability.

It is therefore suggested that a directory of area structure and supportive services is identified and kept collectively.

Please give thought to where this information is going to be kept and who will have access to it.

Immediate area/ward environment

Exercise: Look at your own ward area and consider its geography. Identify the structure and the facilities of the ward. Identify the vulnerable places in your ward; for example, the places where visibility of patients is limited unless staff are in the immediate area, and where equipment is not readily available.

Have you ever thought about the fact that the ward layout may in some respect dictate the organisation of care?

Ward layout tends to be along one of the following designs:

The Nightingale ward

The Bay ward

The Race-track ward

The nucleus ward with various modifications which may create the radial principle.

Various factors have been identified with regard to ward structure that may have implications for ward management:

- *Visibility of patients by nurses and nurses by patients*

- *Concentration of available equipment in parts of the ward*

- *Walking distance between patients and various areas of the ward*

- *The needs of the patient for privacy or solitude.*

If a comparison is done of the layouts it is apparent that the ward manager will need to take the factors of layout and equipment into account.

- *Think where the patients requiring a high dependency of care will be placed*

- *Think where the patients that may require minimal nursing intervention but access to a toilet, will be placed*

- *Think where the confused noisy patient may be placed to create the least disruption to other patients but still be in an area of easy visibility*

- *Think whether the method of staff allocation is suitable for patient and nurse visibility*

- *Remember the walking distance that may be involved for the nurse to travel between her patients*

- *Remember that visual contact may be the single most important influencing factor for over-all satisfaction both for the patient and the nurse.*

The changing scenario of the ward environment

Many changes have and are occurring within patient care some of which have necessitated the movement of the ward. It is therefore important the manager recognises the possibility of the changing venue.

*Compile a list of the essential requirements of your ward in case of movement **but** also identify the improvements that you feel your ward requires now for the benefit of patient care.*

The improvements that you feel are warranted in your area now should be discussed with the appropriate manager and instituted as soon as possible.

So, **be prepared.** Consider your ward and request necessary changes.

Think about:

- *The Health and Safety regulations including Control of Substances Hazardous to Health (COSHH) and cross infection requirements*
- *The fire regulations*
- *The food policy and the kitchen facilities.*

As a ward manager you may need to speak to other people to have clear guidelines especially if your ward is changing in its venue or type of patients.

Remember also your responsibility as a manager to keep abreast of changes and new regulations (competency and code). For example, how have you implemented the lifting regulations required from 1/1/93 Health and Safety Executive (HSE) European Directives (90/269EC).

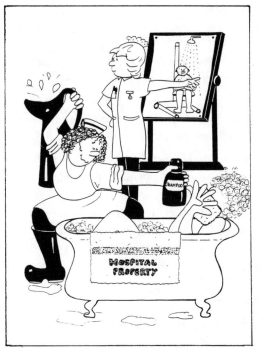

Keep abreast of changes

Gone are the days when we had to lift the patient into the bath because the door was not wide enough for the hoist or the bath was up against the wall so again the hoist could not be used.

The ward environment and the ward visitor

Visitors to the ward encompass all people who enter the ward area whether as patients or for work or social reasons. Hospital policies often cover the requirements involved with visitors (friends or relatives) but general principles of visitors should also be applied to staff members.

Principles to be applied to ward visitors in general:

- *Acknowledge the person*
- *Ascertain their need*

Decide whether:

- *You can meet their need*
- *It is convenient for a relative to see a patient at that precise time*
- *If the doctor can see the patient, you may need to check that the patient is available and not in X-ray or in the toilet*
- *It is a suitable time for repair work to be completed by the works department.*

Following the above then ensure you have *informed, prepared, directed, accompanied,* the person as required.

Make sure that the situation is safe.

Consider:

- *Have measures of infection control been followed?*
- *Have smoking regulations been clarified?*

Also consider whether you have allowed a suitable time period.

Visitors to the ward may include the link teacher for the educational establishment.

The next chapter will look at the link with the educational establishment and the ward learning environment.

References and further reading

Department of Health (1983) *Health of the Nation, targeting practice contributions of nurses, midwives and health visitors.* Department of Health, London

Handy C B (1985) *Understanding Organisations.* Penguin, London

Hunt J W (1992) *Managing people at work.* 3rd Edn. McGraw-Hill Book Company, London

Hyett K (1988) *Nursing Management Handbook.* Churchill Livingstone, Edinburgh

Mersey Regional Health Authority (1991) Workload and skill mix management. *Using Information in Managing the Nursing Resource.* Greenhalgh and Company Limited

Robbins S P (1992) *Essentials of Organisational Behaviour.* 3rd Edn. Prentice Hall International, London

4
The acute ward as a learning environment

Terms used in this section and their definitions

- *Supernumerary*
- *Rostered*
- *Mentor*
- *Supervisor*
- *Assessor*
- *Preceptor*

Supernumerary

A person that exceeds the normal, required or regular number. In the nursing context this means that the ward should be able to function quite adequately without the students. This can be translated in several ways:

- *The students can follow a patient through the different aspects of their care*
- *The students can be part of the functioning team in addition to the normal workforce to gain experience*
- *The students can observe what is happening in a situation.*

Always check the number of hours any student can work. Special duty payments may not be allowed for supernumerary students.

Remember that the student is there to learn and as such should be supervised.

Rostered

A period of allocated work when the student is part of the workforce. It is the time when the student is able to put into practice the experience they have been gaining. In most courses with supernumerary status, a period of rostered service is included during later modules. Please note that the student will still need to be supervised.

Mentor

An individual who has an understanding of the context of the student's learning experience and is selected by the student for the purpose of providing guidance and support (E.N.B. 1994).

Assessor

An appropriately qualified and experienced first level nurse/ midwife/ health visitor who has undertaken preparation to develop skills in facilitating student learning, supervising practice and assessing the student's level of attainment related to the stated outcomes of the programme (E.N.B.1994).

Supervisor

This has been deleted from the glossary of E.N.B. terms (1994) but has been defined as someone who oversees performance ensuring order is maintained at a correct standard. A skilled person helping a person less skilled in a particular activity to achieve competence. The E.N.B sees the roles of supervisor and assessor as being combined to aid the concept of continuous assessment.

Preceptor

An experienced first level nurse/midwife/health visitor who acts as a supporter and colleague for a newly registered practitioner or a practitioner re-entering .

According to the UKCC (1995) the period of preceptorship should average four months, during which the registered practitioner is accountable for their actions. Through mutual negotiation, the practitioner may seek guidance from their preceptor.

Many wards have student nurses working on them as part of the student's education programme. These students are undertaking a variety of courses and many routes are being followed to achieve qualification.

In the authors' experience the following types of students can be found in any one ward.

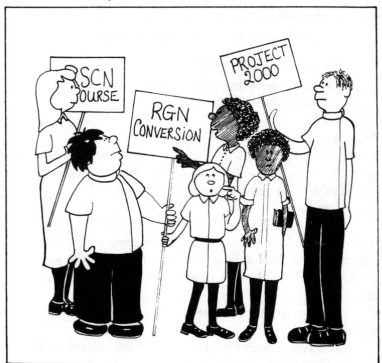

1.   Certificate students

   - *Conversion courses*
   - *Traditional courses*
   - *ENB Pilot scheme courses*

2.   Diploma students

   - *Direct entry midwifery courses*
   - *Non-Project 2000 diploma courses*
   - *Project 2000 courses common foundation +
     branches*
   - *Post registration ENB courses*

3.   Undergraduate students

   - *Regional courses*
   - *Local Higher Education courses*

4.   Health care assistant students

   - *National vocational qualification courses*

5.   Paramedic and medical students

   - *Physiotherapists, occupational therapists,
     radiographers*

Although there may be a wide range of students linked with your ward there are some key principles which can be applied to all of them. Each student will be part of an educational establishment. In this section the Educational Establishment will be the focus of discussion.

The ward will normally have some form of link system with the Educational Establishment. Postal channels will inform of the allocations and there will be a teacher allocated to the ward. This teacher may be a 'lecturer practitioner', 'clinical teacher', 'link nurse teacher'.

For the purpose of this section they will be referred to as the link teacher.

This teacher may have a variety of responsibilities according to their job description. It is important that the ward staff and the teacher build up a working relationship which can be of mutual benefit.

Some aspects of the link teachers role:

- *A representative from the educational establishment facilitating a good working relationship between the educational establishment and the ward*

- *A teacher who can advise, support and assist the staff in their many roles, particularly the roles of mentor/ assessor/ supervisor/ preceptor*

- *A contact who can give an up-to-date picture of what is happening in the educational field*

- *Someone who can help you devise objectives and a philosophy for the ward*

- *Part of a team who will audit and monitor the learning environment*

- *A teacher who can maximise the learning opportunities on the ward for both the staff and the students*

- *Someone who can demonstrate the relevance of the theoretical component of the course to practice, particularly in the realm of assignments which the students have to undertake*

- *An experienced nurse who can help the ward staff support a student who may be experiencing difficulties, by working on the ward or advising the staff of levels of expectation*

- *An advocate for the needs of the patients/ ward/ students in the college of nursing.*

The teaching of nursing has changed considerably over the last few years particularly since the structure has been competency based.

Exercise

Take five minutes to think how different nursing is in your experience from 20 / 10 / 5 / 2 years ago. The further you can go back, the greater the number of changes you will be able to list.

Project 2000 students and others more recently qualified will have more emphasis laid on the value of health in contrast to the healing of illness. Patients are now viewed holistically rather than the *'hernia in bed three'* or *'that sweet old granny who's a bit batty'*.

The following is a list of the sort of subjects a student will now be taught to achieve the competencies (see Appendix 1). Some ideas are added for you to see some of the ways you could link theory to practice and you could use your link teacher to help you translate the course that is taught from your college of nursing.

   Nursing theory and practice

   Physiology

   Sociology

   Psychology

   Health studies

   Professional studies

Nursing theory and practice

Competencies

c)   The use of relevant literature to inform the practice of nursing.

i)   The identification of the needs of patients and clients to enable them to progress from varying degrees of dependence to maximum independence or to a peaceful death.

j)   The ability to devise a plan of care, contribute to its
      implementation and evaluation: and the demonstration of
      the application of the principles of a problem-solving
      approach to the practice of nursing.

As a qualified nurse it is your responsibility to ensure this aspect
of the Nurses Midwives and Health Visitors Act (1979) is carried
out within the framework of the nursing process.

Many nursing models will be taught to the student during a
three year course. The student will need to see how these are
applied in practice.

Consider:

- *Do you* **actually** *use a model on your ward ?*

- *Is the model reflected in your nursing
  documentation?*

- *Does your ward produce care plans which are
  user friendly ?*

- *Are the care plans updated, countersigned and a
  tool which is safe to use ?*

Whilst on the ward the student will need to see and discuss:

- *The basis of the patient assessment carried out
  on your ward*

- *How to identify the patient's 'problems', 'needs'
  or 'self-care deficits' and how to prioritise these*

- *How to plan the care related to the above and
  set goals for the care, whether on a pre-printed
  plan or written for each patient*

- *Specific ways to implement the care according
  to the ward's objectives*

- *Ways by which the results can be evaluated.*

You may consider that many of the student nurses coming to your ward are inept at delivering care. The amount of 'hands on' experience they receive is very limited so they must have as much exposure to excellent care as is possible. They are taught to expect practice to be underpinned by research and you need to be sure that this is so.

Physiology

Competencies

b)   The recognition of common factors which contribute to, and those which adversely affect physical well-being of patients and clients and take appropriate action.

j)   The identification of physical needs of the patient or client.

Many qualified nurses will remember anatomy and physiology. Current thinking in nurse education emphasises physiology and expects the student to learn the relevant anatomy in advance.

The students are taught an understanding of the body's processes. This information is often to a considerable depth but there is a need for the theory to be applied to the practice in the ward situation. Physiology is often taught by a 'systems approach' which sometimes means a student may have difficulty linking the effects of, for example, the implications for renal function if the heart is not functioning adequately.

When a student comes to the ward they need to note the normal and altered physiological responses of the body.

Students can be helped in the following ways:

- *Practice in taking observations and discussing the implications*

- *Assisting in assessing patients so they understand the physiological implications of problems such as pain, pressure sores, malnutrition and wound healing. Wound healing in itself can involve discussing the structure and function of the skin, how the wound heals, the important nutrients in the diet to assist in wound healing, how they are derived from the diet and the body's immune system and the defences against infection*

- *Allowing the student to follow a patient through the operating theatre or X-ray department so that they can see the actual structure that is involved and possibly surrounding structures. For example, they should recognise that abdominal surgery involves the handling of several organs and should recognise the implications of altered nervous system function to the intestines*

- *Getting students to think through why a drug may work in a particular way, or what is the physiology behind a blood transfusion reaction.*

Sociology

Competencies

b) The recognition of common factors which contribute to, and those which adversely affect social well-being of patients and clients and take appropriate action.

d) The appreciation of the influence of social and political factors in relation to health care.

j) The identification of social needs of the patient or client.

Within the subject of sociology the student will study the following range of topics:

- *The constitution of an organisation and its possible structure, especially that of the National Health Service*

- *Social policies which affect health care provision*
- *The definition of a profession and the requirements that constitute acquisition of professional status*
- *The effects and expectations of labelling, illness, the sick role and institutionalisation on an individual.*

When the student comes to the ward they may be able to apply the theory of sociology in the following ways:

- *Discussing the ward structure, its organisation, style of leadership and the expectations of the roles of each member of staff and themselves*
- *Discussing the application of various policies and Acts of Parliament at ward level — for example, the Patients Charter, N.H.S. and Community Care Act*
- *Identifying if a patient is becoming an unpopular patient and discuss how that labelling occurred*
- *Noting the effects of hospitalisation/ institutionalisation on a patient and the keeping of rules and regulations*
- *Assisting the student to identify the patient's social background, their position in the Registrar General's classification and the possible implications on education and the patient's ability to understand the available health services*
- *Being involved in the discharge of patients which may include the setting up of Social Service Support.*

Psychology

Competencies

b) The recognition of common factors which contribute to, and those which adversely affect mental well being of patients and clients and take appropriate action.

f) The use of appropriate communication skills to enable the development of helpful caring relationships with patients and clients and their families and to initiate and conduct therapeutic relationships with patients and clients.

j) The identification of psychological needs of the patient or client: an awareness of values and concepts of individual care.

Psychological theory covers a wide range of topics including personality, attitudes, values, memory, learning and coping mechanisms, including dealing with stress.

When the student comes to the ward they can be helped to apply the knowledge of psychology in the following ways:

- *Learning about themselves in both the way they present themselves and in the way others see them. The student must be given guidance not only on the way they perform physically but in their psychological approach*

- *A difficult area is determining a student's attitude and whether or not it is 'professional'*

- *Helping a student be assertive*

- *Discussing and role modelling various coping mechanisms that they, other members of staff, patients or relatives may use in order to deal with the stressful incidents which may occur*

- *Highlighting these topics in the context of a teaching session on a ward*

- *Allowing the student, under supervision, to practice teaching skills in a safe context*
- *Demonstrating the effects of good communication skills in all aspects of the ward's working life verbally and non-verbally.*

Health studies

Competencies

a)   The identification of the health implications of disease, disability or ageing for the individual, her or his friends and family.

b)   The recognition of common factors which contribute to, and those which adversely affect well-being of patients and clients and take appropriate action.

g)   The identification of health related learning needs of patients and clients, families and friends and to participate in health promotion.

k)   The ability to participate in a multi-professional approach to the care of patients and clients.

l)   The use of the appropriate channel of referral for matters not within her sphere of competence.

The theoretical component for this topic looks at some of the following:

- *Health promotion*
- *Health education*
- *Health maintenance*
- *Health of the Nation*

- *Alternative methods/therapies for relieving stress and maintaining health*

- *Skills required for assessing, planning, implementing and evaluating health related teaching.*

When the student arrives on the ward they will need help applying the theory in the following ways:

- *Identifying pertinent areas of health promotion and health education*

- *Assisting the student to determine lifestyle factors which affect the patient's health*

- *Determining the level of input a patient may need for example, Primary (preventing illness), Secondary (teaching when at risk) and Tertiary (when a problem has occurred)*

- *Discussing programmes of health education already in progress on your ward and allowing the student to participate in these*

- *Identifying any of the Health of the Nation targets which are being tackled*

- *Allowing the student to observe any alternative therapies which may be practised on your ward*

- *Giving the opportunity to practice, under supervision, skills of health teaching*

- *Drawing attention to the different agencies available to help patients.*

Professional studies

Many subjects come under the umbrella of this title. For the purpose of this section, the subjects under discussion will be education, research, ethics, law, professionalism, spirituality and management.

The nurse may be taught 'education' in the form of maths/ study skills/speed reading/appropriate note taking/writing references/library skills/report writing/teaching skills and information technology.

On the ward the student may apply these skills by:

- *Being able to calculate drug and intravenous infusion dosages correctly, and complete fluid charts*

- *Writing accurate nursing records*

- *Teaching patients and colleagues*

- *Applying the skills taught in information technology to the different computerised systems found in a ward area.*

Research

Competency

c)   The use of relevant research to inform the practice of nursing.

Most courses will have a research component to enable the students to read research and apply it appropriately. Normally a research proposal will need to be undertaken at some point. Use your students' knowledge in this respect. No one nurse can know all the research which has been undertaken. Through the research skills the student will have done literature searching, critiquing of literature and then the application through the research proposal.

As previously stated under nursing theory and practice, the student will have been taught to apply research knowledge to practice. It is the qualified nurse's responsibility to ensure that the most up-to-date and research based care is given to the patient, and the student needs access to the relevant information.

Ethics/law/professionalism/ spirituality

The students are given a theoretical basis for each of these subjects.

Ethics

Competency

h)   An understanding of the ethics of health care and of the
     nursing profession and the responsibilities which these
     impose on the nurse's professional practice.

Different principles of ethics, ethical decision making will be
taught and opportunities to discuss ethical problems will be given.
On the ward the student will need:

- *To identify factors within ethical situations*
- *Support for any decision they may have to make.*

They may also need help to come to terms with decisions made
when an ethical dilemma arises.

Law

Competency

e)   An understanding of the requirements of legislation
     relevant to the practice of nursing.

Many educational establishments now give a fairly comprehensive
amount of input regarding legal issues in nursing. This may include
an overview of the legal structure in operation in the relevant part
of the United Kingdom, and an overview of laws affecting nursing
practice.
On the ward a student will need help to identify:

- *Situations in which a legal infringement may*
  take place
- *The nurses role and responsibility to keep within*
  the law.

This may be the ordering, storing, prescribing, and administration of drugs. The safe keeping of patients' property, the safety of all personnel on a ward and the maintenance of confidentiality are other aspects which may be taught.

Professionalism

Competency

e)   An understanding of the requirements of legislation relevant to the practice of nursing.

h)   An understanding of the ethics of health care and of the nursing profession and the responsibilities which these impose on the nurse's professional practice.

Professionalism is discussed in its sociological context and also in application through the UKCC's Standards and advisory booklets. Reference to the Code of Professional Conduct should be expected.

On the ward the student will need to be shown by example

- *How the various UKCC advisory booklets can be applied in practice.*

Spirituality

Competencies

j)   The identification of spiritual needs of the patient or client.

d)   The appreciation of cultural factors in relation to health care.

Spirituality is another subject usually covered and it is often completely associated with religion and possibly death. This subject is covered in a more general sense recognising that many patients have no formal expression to their spirituality.

On the ward a student should be able to:

- *Ask the patient appropriate questions about his/her spiritual needs*

- *Have a knowledge of some of the religious observances a patient may wish to practise.*

Management

Competencies

k)   The ability to function effectively in a team and participate in a multi-professional approach to the care of patients and clients.

m)   The assignment of appropriate duties to others and the supervision, teaching and monitoring of assigned duties.

The final subject the student will need to apply in practice is that of management. This book has hopefully given many ideas. One subject which has not been mentioned in any detail is that of information technology in today's health care. Students are often taught or encouraged to learn the skills of word processing and the use of computers. The application of information technology in the clinical areas needs to be brought to the student's attention so that aspects such as the Data Protection Act (1984) and Access to Medical Records Act (1990) can be applied.

So often the thought of teaching or supervising a student on a course which leads to a higher qualification or a more up to date one can leave the qualified nurse quite nervous and lacking in confidence. It is easy to have negative attitudes towards something which is new and different. It must be remembered that each of us has a unique set of experiences and knowledge. We should work in a team sharing the theoretical and practical knowledge each of us possesses. If you are lacking in knowledge in a particular area there is a golden opportunity for you with PREP and the ENB Higher Award Framework to learn to target your deficit.

Assessment on the ward

Students, like patients need to be assessed before any form of educational programme can take place on the ward. Sometimes it is difficult to remember which student is which, particularly if the uniform is the same or they are wearing a white coat.

Some students are supernumerary, some are rostered and some are just on a visit.

With different agencies negotiating contracts with the hospital authorities there can be confusion with correspondence, 'change lists' and the student who telephones to arrange their own placement. For sheer organisational simplicity, allocate a space – drawer/filing cabinet/box file/correspondence tray – to keep everything together, and let other members of staff know where this is.

Each student will have some range of objectives to fulfil and some form of practical assessment tool. This can range from more traditional 'one-off' assessments through different forms of continuous practical assessment objectives.

The issuing educational establishment will have some form of philosophy to underpin the objectives.

Exercise

Discover the philosphy (philosophies) that underpin the objectives you use.

An example of steps towards practical assessment achievement

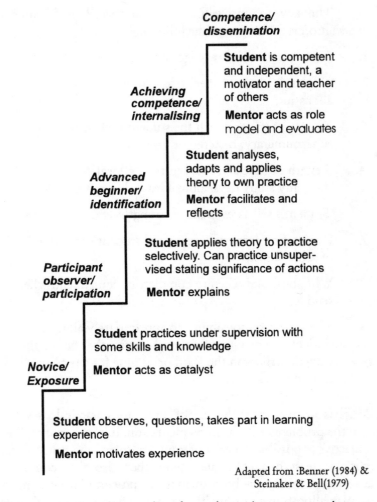

**Competence/
dissemination**

Student is competent
and independent, a
motivator and teacher
of others

Mentor acts as role
model and evaluates

*Achieving
competence/
internalising*

Student analyses,
adapts and applies
theory to own practice

Mentor facilitates and
reflects

*Advanced
beginner/
identification*

Student applies theory to practice
selectively. Can practice unsuper-
vised stating significance of actions

Mentor explains

*Participant
observer/
participation*

Student practices under supervision with
some skills and knowledge

Mentor acts as catalyst

*Novice/
Exposure*

Student observes, questions, takes part in learning
experience

Mentor motivates experience

Adapted from :Benner (1984) &
Steinaker & Bell(1979)

These steps, using the wording from the various taxonomies, can
be applied to any skill. The focus must be identified.

The document may be organised under a variety of focal sections, eg problem solving approach or the subject heading listed earlier.

The key to unravelling the educational establishment's expectation is to determine the following:

1. Student's prior knowledge and experience.

2. Student's level of experience — now and at end of allocation.

3. The status under which the student will work — eg supernumerary, rostered or visit.

4. Length of time and continuity of allocation — eg are there any study days/annual leave during this time?

5. Student's self assessment of strengths and weaknesses.

6. Expectation from document and student's expected level of achievement.

7. Who, how and when to complete document and where to send it.

8. The ward's responsibility to appropriately allocate a student to a qualified first level nurse either before the student arrives on the ward or in time for the counselling session to take place.

Much is written on the theories of continuous practical assessment and the problems with its implementation. It is important to be as objective as possible. Check out your comments about any student with at least one colleague. Remember also that continuous assessment must have both **formative** and **summative** elements, so plan allocation accordingly. Try not to be too egocentric when dealing with student assessments. It is only too easy to say, 'in my day I had a practical room assessment and that was good enough for me', or for those not so long in the tooth , 'our continuous practical assessment document was much easier to fill in than this one!' As always, **practice makes perfect.**

The assessment is important to the student and will be their only opportunity to gain experience and confidence and demonstrate that they are achieving the competencies that are required. You may act as mentor/ assessor/ preceptor/ supervisor to many students, but it must be a new relationship with each student.

To help with your role within the assessment field, you must conform with the UKCC's expectations and acquire the suitable preparation for the role of mentor / assessor / preceptor / supervisor in the clinical environment.

Often in practice the roles of mentor/ assessor/ preceptor/ supervisor seem to merge into one. For the purpose of this section on qualities of a mentor/assessor/supervisor/preceptor the term advisor will be used to indicate the collective qualities of the four roles. The reader is recommended to review the definitions of the role as stated on pages 66-67.

What are the skills and attitudes you need to possess to undertake this role?

There are four key concepts (adapted from Barber and Norman 1987):

- **Supportive role** — *empathetic and approachable, recognising and tackling issues potentially and actually causing stress reduction*

- **Educational role** — *equipping nurses with necessary knowledge and skills, answering how and why questions*

- **Managerial role** — *assessing strengths and weaknesses, planning allocation and evaluation of work*

- **Catalyst role** — *developing personal awareness, confidence and self esteem. Role model demonstrating appropriate attitudes.*

Your College of Nursing will normally have a policy relating to the above roles and this will include information such as:

- *Who can be an advisor*

- *The specified number of times in any one week that this person would work with a student*

- *Timing of each part of the assessment such as initial or preliminary assessment / counselling, midway or ongoing assessment / counselling, final or concluding assessment / counselling*

- *What to do in the event of; a problem student, a problem member of qualified staff, a problem with the achievement of objectives.*

This last situation may stem from a projected ward closure or reduction in the number of patients and the suitability of the clinical area.

The good advisor guide

1. Welcome the student to the ward.
    Show them round and give them opportunity to ask questions.
    Indicate important aspects of your ward eg:

    - *Fire escapes, fire extinguishers, fire alarms*

    - *Resuscitation equipment, drug cupboard/ trolley*

    - *Location of the telephone*

    - *Location and general contents of documents on the ward such as Health and Safety folder and Nursing Procedures folder*

    - *Ward philosophy and objectives*

    - *Staff names, duty rotas and general idiosyncrasies.*

2. Discuss the experiences available to the student on the ward and determine the students:

   - *Strengths and weaknesses*
   - *What they must achieve on the ward*
   - *Individual needs.*

3. Be a positive role model

   - *Be patient*
   - *Demonstrate good communication, counselling and interpersonal skill.*

Helpful qualities of an advisor

- *Being prepared for student's arrival on ward*
- *Willingness to answer questions and offer explanations*
- *Interest in students and a respect for them*
- *Giving encouragement and praise*
- *Giving information about progress*
- *Giving constructive criticism*
- *An appropriate sense of humour*
- *A pleasant voice*
- *Being available when needed*
- *Giving appropriate supervision*
- *Displaying confidence in own and student's abilities.*

Hindering qualities of an advisor

- *Domineering behaviour*
- *Inconsistency*
- *Sarcasm*
- *Acting in a superior manner*

- *Belittling students*
- *Correcting students in the presence of others*
- *Supervising too closely*
- *Emphasising mistakes and weaknesses*
- *Ignoring student*
- *Incorrect or late completion of assessment documents.*

With all the many demands on the time of the ward staff it is often difficult to remember the individual needs of the students. A 'white board' or notice board listing who was mentor to whom and when pertinent assessments were due could facilitate everyone's memory. The board could also include the specific learning objectives each student should achieve on your ward.

This board should never substitute for the personal contact between the two individuals and time and a private space should be set aside for the key assessment points and also for ongoing progress reports.

Never leave it to an assessment point to tell a student that their work is poor, as they will invariably not have enough time to improve.

Feedback should be given **at the time** and not several days / weeks later. Feedback, whether negative or positive, about a student's practice should be given as near to the time of occurrence as possible. It is rarely easy to tell a student that their work is not of an acceptable standard. It must be done in a discreet manner but sufficiently clearly and with the relevant input and support to enable that particular student to improve.

Praise for good work done is something that is forgotten on a busy day. This can make such a difference to anybody and does wonders for confidence, self-esteem and the motivation highlighted earlier in chapter two. Do not let praise slip off the tongue in a glib manner though, as this can sound rather hollow and not encourage the individual as it should.

It is important to remember at this point that the ward team

must fulfil it's responsibility to the student. As a manager it is also
your responsibility to ensure that the student is suitably supervised
and that the notion of accountability regarding the student's work
is understood.

The UKCC's (1992) Code of Professional Conduct states:

> *As a registered nurse, midwife or health visitor, you
> are personally accountable for your practice and, in
> the exercise of your professional accountability,*
> **must:**
>
> *Clause 1. Act always in such a manner as to promote
> and safeguard the interests and well-being of patients
> and clients*
>
> *Clause 2. Ensure that no action or omission on your
> part, or within your sphere of responsibility, is
> detrimental to the interests, condition or safety of
> patients and clients*
>
> *Clause 3. Maintain and improve your professional
> knowledge and competence*
>
> *Clause 4. Acknowledge any limitations in your
> knowledge and competence and decline any duties or
> responsibilities unless able to perform them in a safe
> and skilled manner*
>
> *Clause 14. Assist professional colleagues, in the context
> of your own knowledge, experience and sphere of
> responsibility, to develop their professional competence,
> and assist others in the health care team...to contribute
> safely and to a degree appropriate to their roles*

The organisation of the learning environment

The whole concept of the ward learning environment has been left to last.

Questions you may ask about the organisation of your ward learning environment are:

1. What are the learning opportunities on the ward ?

2. Who or what are barriers to learning ?

3. How do the staff tackle teaching and learning on the ward ?

4. Is there an organised framework ?

5. Do you plan teaching/supervision or does it just 'happen'?

A useful exercise would be to answer these questions and then, if there are areas which are not satisfactory, decide what are you going to do about them.

Ideas:

1. Devise objectives to be achieved on your ward.

2. Barriers could include:
   - *Unwillingness to answer questions*
   - *Poorly structured routine*
   - *Unapproachable staff*
   - *Students lacking assertive skills*
   - *The ward being too busy*

3. Teaching can be informal and 'as you go along' rather than sitting down 'in a huddle' but it still needs to be planned.

4. As mentioned earlier a board for information regarding advisors could be extended to include subject areas for teaching. Consider the geography of the ward, the

overlap of your staff and time for teaching, group size, privacy and confidentiality when planning your teaching.

If you are the ward manager be aware that you hold the key to the ward learning environment. As the ward manager identify how effectively you control the ward learning environment.

If you are a staff nurse or a student consider — how you can positively influence the ward's learning environment?

In either case, are **you** one of the barriers to learning? Refer back to the good advisor guide as the barriers are similar.

Teaching is an important facet of management in an acute ward.

Competency

> m) 'the assignment of appropriate duties to others and the supervision, teaching and monitoring of assigned duties'

Our prime responsibility as nurses is the care of the patients but a well organised and well prepared and integrated staff team comes second. We are all learners.

What would you do in the following situations?

1. Your ward evaluates poorly under the heading of 'Ward learning environment stimulated me to learn' section. What steps could you take to rectify this stated problem?

2. Your qualified staff consist of:

   - *1 x G grade — yourself*

   - *1 x F grade — going on maternity leave in 2 weeks*

   - *2 x E grades — one gave 4 week's notice last week*

- *4 x D grade —2 starting (newly qualified) next week*

- *1 x C grade — starting conversion course in 2 weeks.*

You have planned for the F and C grades being off the ward but you were unaware of the E grade's imminent departure. What do you do about the 2 first ward supernumerary students who start on the ward on Monday?

3.   A third year rostered student is not achieving their objectives on the ward. They say this is the first allocation they have been on where they have not done well. *'My mentor is useless,'* they moan. As the ward manager what do you do?

4.   Your ward is constantly busy. You have been qualified 3 months and are (without preparation) acting as a mentor for two first year students. You find the whole situation quite overwhelming but recognise that all the staff are similarly pressurised. How might you deal with the problem?

5.   You are the F grade on an acute medical ward where there is little overlap time in the afternoon between shifts. Your manager has asked you to revamp the teaching strategy for your ward. What could you do?

6.   A student writes in their evaluation of the ward that they think your ward was the best they had worked on so far. What would you do?

Suggested tactics:

1.
- *Talk to your link teacher and ask for more details if they are available, also ask for some ideas for improvement*

- *Ask the students currently on the ward what they think*

- *Discuss the problem with the staff and seek their solutions*

- *Get a volunteer nominee to be responsible for this aspect of the ward and give that individual support and encouragement*

- *Review the situation in 3 months time and check the next set of evaluation documents for improvement*

2.
- *You need to contact the educational establishment and state your situation. They may be able to re-allocate the students although it may be difficult*

- *Contact your nursing officer or equivalent and ask for support and practical help in the way of permanent 'bank' nurses pending a new appointment*

- *Follow protocol to close beds, if pertinent*

- *Document all your actions bearing in mind clauses 4, 11, 12 and 13 of the Code of Professional Conduct (1992)*

3.
- *Discuss with the student the exact nature of their complaint*

- *Discuss with the advisor the importance and extent of their role, supporting them as much as possible*

- *Inform the link teacher and possibly the students' personal teacher of the problem and discuss solutions*

- *Work out with the advisor and student a plan for the remaining time on the ward to maximise the student's opportunities*

4.
- *You are a very junior staff nurse and need the support of the more senior qualified staff on your ward*
- *Inform them of your problem*
- *Talk to the link teacher and ask for advice and support in dealing with your students*
- *Determine how you will prioritise your work to get everything done to the highest standard*
- *Gain a place on a recognised teaching and/or assessing course, such as the E.N.B. 998 course in order to prepare yourself*
- *With the next group of students perhaps ask for a break, only take one student or share two students between you and another more senior staff nurse*

5.
- *Discuss this situation with the rest of the staff as you will need their co-operation*
- *Ask the student what they want covered. Talk to the link teacher and ask them to assist in the programme*
- *Determine the objectives for your teaching and the topics you hope to cover. Decide which will be taught formally /informally*
- *Plan an outline programme which is achievable and set a start date.* **Start — then evaluate**

6.
- *Let the staff know. Do not be complacent*

Conclusion

Implicit in the text has been the sense that the person who acts as the manager will be where the buck stops. This is not necessarily the case. The ward team consists of staff that are responsible in their own rights.

Everyone has their own responsibilities.

The ward manager, as described, the staff nurses to the team, the students for their objectives and the care assistants for their National Vocational Qualifications. This needs to be recognised for the harmony of the team. However the ward manager must manage the team of staff.

The complexities of management are difficult to include in one book. We have attempted to look at some of the aspects of management and link them to the position of a ward manager. We have tried to give some workable exercises that can either be done in advance, or whilst learning about ward management, or can act as a ready guide to some situations whilst holding the position of a ward manager.

We especially want to emphasise the section of examining yourself as a leader and recognising the effect that your personality and management style can have on the team in which you work. An interesting question to ask yourself now or in the future is: *'How will the ward run in my absence?'*

Often the sign of a good manager is the fact that the ward will run well in your absence. **Think about it!**

The ward will run well because you will have helped the staff to see their roles and to know how to perform them independently. Be proud of this fact.

Work towards a staff who can manage without you.

This will not mean that you will no longer have a position in the team, but that you have developed your team. In order to develop your team you need to spend time developing yourself. There are a wealth of courses on management, nursing, research and changes in nursing.

Ensure you attempt to keep yourself up to date and that you communicate this information to the ward team. This in itself may be a full-time job at present with the multitude of changes that are occurring. However, remember that you can not do this all yourself. Involve the ward team and learn from the staff that you have on the ward.

There are so many aspects to consider in management, we hope this book can guide you through some of them and that you will take the opportunity to do further reading to enhance your skills.

References and further reading

Barber P & Norman I (1987) Skills in Supervision. *Nurs Times*, **Jan 14,** 56-57

Benner P (1984) *From Novice to Expert*. Addison-Wesley, California

Dimond B (1993) *Patients' Rights, Responsibilities and the Nurse.* Tingle J (Ed). Quay Books, Mark Allen Publishing Ltd, Dinton, Salisbury

ENB (1994) Changes to regulations and guidelines for the approval of institutions and courses. *ENB News* **14**

Steinaker N & Bell M (1979) *Experiential Taxonomy.* Academic Press, New York

Tschudin V (1993) *Ethics: Nurses and Patients.* Scutari Press, London

UKCC (1992) *Code of Professional Conduct.* UKCC, London

UKCC (1995) Registrar's Letter 03/95 *The Council's position concerning a period of support and preceptorship* Annex 1. UKCC, London

Appendix 1

Rule 18a

The stated professional competencies in Nursing, Midwifery and Health Visitors Rules Approval Order 1989 No 1456 (September 1989)

a. The identification of the social and health implications of pregnancy and child bearing, physical and mental handicap, disease, disability, or ageing for the individual, her or his friends, family and community

b. The recognition of common factors which contribute to, and those which adversely affect, physical, mental and social well-being of patients and clients and take appropriate action

c. The use of relevant literature and research to inform the practice of nursing

d. The appreciation of the influence of social, political and cultural factors in relation to health care

e. An understanding of the requirements of legislation relevant to the practice of nursing

f. The use of appropriate communication skills to enable the development of helpful caring relationships with patients and clients and their families and friends, and to initiate and conduct relationships with patients and clients

g. The identification of health related learning needs of patients and clients, families and friends and to participate in health promotion

h. An understanding of the ethics of health care and of the nursing profession and the responsibility which these impose on the nurse's professional practice

i.   The identification of the needs of patients and clients to
        enable them to progress from varying degrees of
        dependence to maximum independence, or to a peaceful
        death

j.   The identification of physical, psychological, social and
        spiritual needs of the patients or client; and awareness of
        values and concepts of individual care; the ability to devise
        a plan of care, contribute to its implementation and
        evaluation; and the demonstration of a problem-solving
        approach to the care of patients and clients

k.   The ability to function effectively in a team and
        participate in a multi-professional approach to the care of
        patients and clients

l.   The use of the appropriate channel of referral for matters
        not within her sphere of competence

m.   The assignment of appropriate duties to others and the
        supervision, teaching and monitoring of assigned duties

Index

A
Accountability 21
Assessment 82
Assessor 66
Attitudes 20
Audit 51
B
Behavioural theory 14
C
Care
direct 6
indirect 5, 6
Change 58
Code of Professional
  Conduct 23, 89
Communication 28
Competence 21
Control 27
D
Decision making 44
Delegation 45
Direct care 6
Documentation 43
Duty rotas 37
E
Educational audit 51
Environment
hospital 57
learning 65, 90
ward 58
Evaluation 50
Evaluator 49
G
Goal
achievement 52
setting 52

H
Health studies 76
Hospital environment 57
I
Implementation 46
Indirect care 5,6
J
Job
achievement 47
satisfaction 47
K
Knowledge19
L
Law 79
Leadership12
behavioural theory 14
characteristics 16
contingency theory 14
trait theory 13
Learning environment 65
Link teacher 68, 69
M
Management
self 3
Manager
needs 1
as a leader 20
for students 81
Mentor 66
Motivation 47
staff 47
N
Named nurse 42
Needs
patients 6
Negotiation 33

Nursing
  practise 70
  theory 42
O
Organisational
  change 53
  structure 23
P
Patient
  care 36, 37
  needs 6
  satisfaction 51
Philosophy 26
Physiology 72
Planning 35
Preceptor 67
Primary nursing 41
Professional studies 77
Professionalism 80
Psychology 75
R
Responsibility 21
Role 1
Rules and Regulations 25
S
Skills 19
Sociology 73
Spirituality 80
Staff
  appraisal 50
  record 39
Students 65
  rostered 66
  supernumerary 65
Supervisor 66

T
Team nursing 41
Teacher 69
Time
  wasting 35
  management 3
Trait theory 13
U
Use of time 3
V
Values 73
  clarification 7
Visitors 61
W
Ward 40
  layout 58
  learning environment 65
  visitors 61